CANCER

Traditional
and
New Concepts

Compiled
by
Hanna Kroeger, Ms.D
Minister
of the Chapel of Miracles

This book is written in memory of
Prof. Brauchle, M.D., Dresden.

I sincerely wish that the knowledge of this genius will help you and your beloved ones.

That his torch will kindle and save our nation from the scorch of Cancer and Leukemia.

Prof. Brauchle died in the flames of Dresden, while carrying leukemia stricken children to safety.

ISBN: 1-883713-06-4

CONTENTS

INTRODUCTION

CANCER

The word "Cancer" has such a terrible sound. It is a death sentence in six letters. It is an end of all your dreams. It ruins your family. It ruins springtime and the fall. You can't see the beauty of the flowers any longer, nor the sky with the sailing clouds. The helping hand you push away, because you gave in to six small letters, "cancer." The "C" is twice in this word, just to make it sharp and pointed, irritating and hurting. With its hooks, it penetrates your mind, and like a fish hook in your flesh, this hook cannot be pulled out of your mind easily. It sticks in your mind—"cancer, I have cancer."

Cancer has become one of the most common diseases in America. Every third person has it, and statistics go as far as to say every second person has it. We should be used to hearing the word "cancer" without fear. But, instead, the fear phantom increases with every case diagnosed. This fear syndrome is paralyzing to our inborn defense mechanism. We just give in. Like a mouse is paralyzed for fear when a snake comes close, so, most of us are paralyzed when the verdict is given that *you* have cancer.

We go to our desks and start cleaning out. We put our estates and affairs in order. In our minds, we say good-bye to all plans and dreams we have for the future. And we retreat into a shell that screams, "Don't touch me, I am doomed."

If this happens to *you*, turn around and uplift your life. Go to the dress shop and spend some money on a pink or rose-colored dress, and then get fitted for some high-heeled shoes. Know that you can overcome your resentments and your fear syndrome.

Take a mild, herbal sleeping pill until you are over the first shock. Then start creating your life all over again, new and beautiful.

In every case, when your health has deteriorated to the point of diagnosis, you belong under the guidance of a physician. Besides that, you cannot go on undermining your health with all the wrong-doings you have been doing over the years. Rebuilding your health is your problem, not your physician's. The physician helps you to eliminate illness, but you, and you alone, can rebuild your health.

Health is the most precious possession you, personally, can have. You cannot buy it, you have to work at it. You have to sacrifice for it. Health is your heritage, your freedom from illness. Just as the citizens of a nation have to work and sacrifice for the precious gift of freedom, to hold it and keep it, so the individual has to work on the precious heritage of freedom from illness. You work on it by educating yourself, changing your diet and life-style, changing your outlook to see the purpose of life and by believing in the universal law that "as a man soweth, so will he reap."

CANCER

Traditional Concepts

TRADITIONAL CONCEPTS

DIFFERENT THEORIES ON CANCER

Theory I

Cancer is a disease of fermentation and oxygen deficiency.

According to Nobel Laureate, Dr. Otto Warburg, "The prime cause of cancer is the replacement of the respiration of oxygen in normal body cells by a fermentation of sugar." Dr. Warburg adds that cells that aren't able to derive the oxygen and nutrients essential to energy production can only do *one* thing: *SWITCH OVER TO SUGAR FERMENTATION, OR DIE!!* Dr. Warburg won the Nobel prize for his discovery that cancer is a disease of defective cellular respiration. He has shown that cancer cells generate an abundance of lactic acid because of this partial anaerobic glycosis. In short, Dr. Warburg says cancer is caused by the lack of oxygen at the cellular level.

Theory II

Immune Systems Dysfunction

Science has known for years that cancer patients have a weakened immune system and that a healthy immune system has the ability to destroy DNA damaged cells.

Dr's. Stephen Levine and Parris Kidd have identified this defense system and the cell's ability to adapt to oxidative stress through the glutathione cycle. All sorts of chemicals create free radicals, including endocrine hormones that circulate as a result of stress. These free radicals can stretch the capabilities of the antioxidant defense system to the limit and ultimately render it defenseless if vital nutrients aren't replaced. Before this happens those doctors have found that the antioxidant defense system fails in an attempt to adapt to increased utilization of key nutrients. This causes uncontrolled free radical damage with its cross linking, immune dysfunction and chemical hypersensitivity.

Dr. Hans Nieper, M.D., offers this refreshing approach to repair the immune system:

1 activation of the thymus function
2 activating the immune system
3 activating the enzymatic action of the pancreas

Dr. Nieper gives trypsin bromalain chymotrypsin therapy for thymus gland. Also:

    zinc orotate
    calcium orotate
    magnesium orotate

Dr. Nieper says that protein has to be digested and that the protein layer around the cancer cell has to be broken down. He points out when the magnesium level in the blood gets down it shows *immune system fatigue*. Dr. Nieper says that all people with cancer involvement need 200,000 units of Vitamin A. The best source is seven ounces of carrot juice, three to four times a day. One tablespoon of whipped cream should be added.

Immune System Enhancer

This is a new approach and it works. It is not my idea. The only claim I can make is that I worked on it until it was perfected.

Crystal Laser is a conditioned light beam that you point toward your thymus gland.

This Crystal Laser gives you:

1 A positive attitude towards life.
2 It strengthens the power of positive thinking.
3 It strengthens the immune system.
4 When the thymus gland and immune system are strengthened, flu, colds, and viral infections will be lessened or eliminated.

It is documented that the use of sodium fluoride in toothpaste or water will influence the immune system to a standstill.

Theory III

Faulty Cell Division

Until he was in his late teens, Albert Szent-Györgyi's family thought he was retarded. But he went on to become one of the world's most honored scientists. Now, at the age of eighty-three and after years of research, he has evolved a theory which may solve the deadly mystery of cancer. Dr. Szent-Györgyi calls his discovery the "electronic theory of cancer." It is based on understanding how cells divide and how this process goes wrong to produce wildly dividing and growing "sick" cells—cancer. Because electrons make cells move, they are the key to understanding cell division. Unlike other cancer researchers who are concentrating on the cause of the disease—there are many causes, from viruses to food additives—Dr. Szent-Györgyi focuses on the cell. "You cannot cure what you do not understand. To fix and automobile engine, first you must know how it works," he says. While enormously complex in detail, in essence, his theory is simple. It is based on how cells grow. Cancer is a distortion of this growth, or wild, uncontrolled division of cells. Division is movement; the agent of movement is the electron. Cells are constantly moving between two states. One is a state of proliferation or division. The other is a resting state. When a cell gets stuck in the first proliferating state, as it will if its electronic moving system is out of order, it will divide uncontrollably and the result will be a cancerous growth. "What makes the cell pathological is that it cannot find its way back to the resting state," Dr. Szent-Györgyi says. If a way can be found to introduce electronic mobility into a cancerous cell to move it out of the wild growth state and into the resting state, it could be the eventual answer to cure or prevention of the disease.

In his address at the Boston University School of Medicine Symposium, Dr. Szent-Györgyi dramatically demonstrated a key element in his theory—that certain proteins can carry electrons. He showed a test tube with a yellow liquid, the color indicating that it was not a "semi-conductor" of electrons. But then he showed a second tube. It was an identical liquid, but the color had been changed, by adding a chemical solution, to a dark, opaque red. Some proteins then are semi-conductors.

"The human body," Dr. Szent-Györgyi says, "is a better machine than we think. It is only when we treat it badly that it fails. Benefits from vitamins are not known for perhaps years after we start taking them," he says, "and then we do not know why we feel good."

Another reason for his hearty old age is that he loves his work—research—and the fight against cancer gives him a strong opponent. It has made him, he says, a "happy man."

Theory IV

Cancer is a Fat-Protein problem

Dr. Hedwig Budwig has a different approach to cancer. She said cancer is a fat-protein problem. Dr. Budwig is the world's leading expert on the therapeutic uses of oils, especially flaxseed oil, also called linseed oil.

She recommends oils and cottage cheese to all her cancer cases with phenomenal results. For years I wondered why such a simple remedy can have such super outstanding results.

I learned that with this formula the body can make its own interferon. What are interferons? Interferons are proteins which are manufactured in the cells when the human body is under attack of fungi or viruses. Interferons "interfere" with the ability of both fungi and viruses to multiply in the body.

There seems to be several interferon proteins. The most outstanding is Interleukin-2-. This particular one is used in kidney tumors and in the management of brain tumors. It also seems to depress the formation of new tumors through metastasis. In fact interferon and Interleukin-2- is a weapon against cancer.

Dr. Budwig registers outstanding results in the management of cancer with the use of her formula of "cottage cheese and oil." This formula provides the body with fuel to make its own interferon and its own Interleukin-2-.

This also is the best prevention against cancer in general. Make one of her recipes twice a week and you will be blessed. Here are some recipes which are tasty and helpful.

5 tablespoons of oil as almond oil
or apricot oil
or walnut oil
(Dr. Budwig uses flaxseed oil)

This formula makes interferon in your body. Interferon is needed to combat cancer. In fact, interferon is made in the laboratories and you need 10 bottles of it at $300 for each bottle.

Dr. Budwig said: "Cancer patients have to eat and starve the tumors." She takes raw cottage cheese called "quark" and adds cold pressed oils to it. With this the starved cells are supplied with an oxygen rich product. Even though they never met, her findings coincide with Dr. Szent-Györgyi's research.

Both precious physicians say that certain proteins can carry electrons which are vital for the health of the starving cells. With raw oil Dr. Budwig adds another important factor, "Vitamin F," which also becomes an oxygen carrier to the starving cells.

Foundation Recipe

Put in blender or mix thoroughly by hand:
   1 cup cottage cheese
   2 tablespoons walnut or almond oil

This mixture is the foundation recipe and can be varied.

A)   Add finely grated horseradish. Serve with potatoes, buckwheat, and/or stewed carrots.
B)   To foundation recipe, add spices, such as finely cut parsley, celery, or paprika.
C)   To foundation recipe add: tomatoes or tomato puree to taste. This is very delicious with rice, bulgur, or rye bread.
D)   To foundation recipe add: chives, onion, parsley (finely cut) or paprika (finely cut)
E)   Make a colored surprise by adding to one part of cream cheese, tomato puree, or beets, a second part color with greens such as spinach, and a third part color with egg yolk. Arrange nicely and decorate with cucumber, tomatoes, radishes, etc.
F)   Heap the foundation recipe on lettuce leaves and top with a peach or apricot.
G)   As a dessert, use the cream cheese sweetened with honey. Add a banana, a grated apple and some oatflakes on top.
H)   To cottage cheese mixture add: honey, filberts, walnuts, almonds, all finely cut. Do not use peanuts. This is terrific for the center of a variety fruit plate. It is a whole meal!
I)   Make a little basket of the orange by scraping the inside out and adding honey to the foundation recipe. For parties, fill orange-basket with sweetened recipe.
J)   Use foundation recipe as a salad dressing. Thin with sour milk or thin cream. Add: tarragon, parsley, paprika, rosemary or any herb or spice. Add: vegetable salt and a little lemon juice and more oil. It tastes delicious.
K)   The above salad dressing goes well with: dandelion leaves, endive or white cabbage. Wild roses can be added to any salad. Cut them just before they are in full bloom.

These recipes are terrific to eliminate scar tissue.

CANCER

New Concepts

CANCER

THE NEW CONCEPT

We live in exciting times; we are beginning to understand disease at the molecular level.

New Concept No. I

Cancer is a fungus

55 years ago, I was working and studying in Professor Dr. Brauchle's Hospital for Natural Healing. In one of the professor's lectures he gave to nurses and physicians he said: "Cancer is undoubtedly a fungus. There are several fungi which can attack the human body. Cancer is a type that clusters and makes metastasis. In nature, mushrooms live and prefer decayed matter. You find mushrooms around rotten tree stems, neglected meadows, in the woods and muddy, rotten leaves."

In the human body, cancer fungus will grow as in nature in decaying matter.

a)   in an unhealthy colon
b)   chemical additives to food and drink
c)   improper care of all body functions
d)   stress
e)   wrong food combination
f)   negative mental attitude

With this theory that cancer is a fungus which grows in decaying matter we have to look around and find out

1)   What additives are stored in my body?
2)   Which negative mental attitude do I harbor?
3)   Which foods are good for me?
4)   Which food combinations are right for me?
5)   What parasites have nested in me?

The second question is: What can be done to kill the fungus?

Chemotherapy is designed to kill the fungus and I, working with herbs, suggest that you add our God given herbs to whatever your physician suggests.

Over the years I collected all kinds of herb formulas from various healers used over many centuries. All of them are designed to halt the fungus growth, to diminish the size of the tumor, and to strengthen the system in order to bring back the health of the individual.

11

Self Examination for Fungus Cancer

According to Michael Renny: "If the cancer incidents continue to grow as they have been in the last decade, it will be a matter of extinguishing the human race. Cancer can extinguish mankind as the prehistoric catastrophes have extinguished the dinosaur."

Charles Eliot Perkins said: "Cancer is a profound morbid pathological condition of the entire body and is not confined to local malignant growth."

Self-examination taught in England and Denmark:

Sterilize a pin. Prick one finger tip. When the blood comes with a pearl, you are healthy, when it smears, change your diet and lifestyle. When the drop runs and more than several drops come out from one prick in a thin stream, have an examination by a physician, change your diet, get well quickly, and thank God for this knowledge.

The following method which is taught in America is a tremendous breakthrough in detecting oncoming cancer 2 years before a tumor is formed.

Take the first morning urine in a celluloid cup. (Not a foam cup). Cover it with one layer of toilet paper and place it in a dark place. In the evening set the celluloid cup in your refrigerator (lowest shelf). Secure it so that no one will disturb it. The next morning pour out the urine. Where air and urine touched, there will be a fatty waxy ring in the cup if fungus cancer is present in your system.

Examine yourself every six months.

Herbs in the Management of Fungus Cancer

The Indians are known to have very little cancer. So, I investigated it. It is not the diet because they eat more white sugar and more white bread than any other members of the American continent. But they know Herbs and they are the best herbalists.

The Indians gathered the following Herbs and made a tea out of it:

yellow dock
cramp bark
yarrow
plantain
tansy
milkweed
tobacco*

Milkweed is a North American herb called bloodhoney that is not found in other parts of the world and milkweed is very dear to the Indians. So is tobacco very dear to them and they offer it to their deity. Another tribe took:

alfalfa seed
blessed thistle
golden seal root**

Both these 2 herb formulas taken together shows relief to a fungus-ridden body.

All Indian tribes are aware that cancer victims have parasites and they make sure that these scavengers are removed. They use different kinds of herbs. One Indian lady told me, "Mother cancer in bowels, daughter cancer somewhere else." You have to know that American Indians are born with the 6th sense open clair-voyant, clair-audiant. We have to acquire this through long hours of dedication and meditation.

The Indian observations are so accurate. The Herbs they use are Anti-fungus, not poisonous to the body, only to the fungus.

* Blood Toner
**Foon Goos

13

AN AMERICAN INDIAN HEALING METHOD

FOR FUNGUS CANCER

I had the unbelievable fortune to see Ameri-Indians heal cancer.

They also heal their tumor patients with stones and I found out that they are magnetic stones. They do the following:

The loadstones—magnetic stones are hit with one stroke "to make them active." The person is laid on a cot on the floor. The stones are placed around the person while the Indians make sure that the part that is hit comes close to the body. They place one stone to the head, one on each side of the body and one on the inside of each foot.

A ceremony starts with sage and feathers, with dancing and asking the Great Spirits to remove all dark forces attached to the body. All night the person has to lay like this. They said they have to lay there 3–4 nights as demonstrated. By looking closer I found that it is the Northpole, the negative side, that came close to the body, and they said that the negative tumor is influenced by it.

We do not have loadstones but we have magnets. Why should we not use them? Place Goo Gauss magnets around the body so that the north side, the negative side, touches the body as the Indians do. It takes only 47 hours of treatments to influence the negative tumor. We could try couldn't we?

We also could try antifungal herbs and herb mixtures as the Indians showed us. What harm could be done? Absolutely no harm. These herbs are safe particularly in the minute amounts they are used.

How to Place Magnets

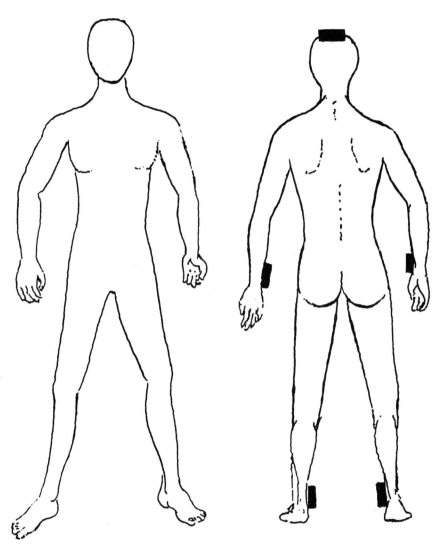

Northside to body

Quaw Bark

Quaw Bark is the inner bark of an American tree. The American Indians used it for centuries to enhance the healing power of their mixtures. Quaw Bark has the same healing property that has been documented in Brazilian Pau D'Arco. When grown in America, we can utilize its vibration readily.

This bark is used as an anti-fungal and for fighting viral infections as well as having claims to giving strength, stamina, endurance and building the immune system.

Asparagus

"Eating cooked asparagus overcame proven cases of cancer," declared Karl B. Lutz, biochemist, in a letter published in Prevention Magazine. Use fresh, steamed asparagus, or asparagus canned without pesticides or preservatives, from Health Food Stores, Green Giant or Stokeley. Never use raw asparagus. Blend in blender at high speed, he advised. Eat four full Tbsp. of asparagus twice daily, morning and evening, hot or cold. The patients usually show improvement in 2 to 4 weeks, he said, and he asked that all who try it, send him a report.

Here is one report. A gentleman about 76 years of age developed cauliflower cancer on the ears which appeared thick, crusted and white in color. He was scheduled for surgery but decided to give asparagus a try. In 3 weeks all of it was gone. Pink, healed, amazing.

Concord Grapes/Grape Juice

Concord grapes and Concord grape juice also are known to work against the fungus. If you do not like it soak dark raisins (currants are best) and drink the juice and eat the soaked raisins.

New Concept No. II

Retro-Virus — The New Comer

Retroviruses are RNA viruses. They are smaller than DNA viruses and they lump together in geometrical patterns. Retroviruses are originally found in animals such as mice and apes. They are a common virus to these creatures and one that does not hurt them. However, when found in humans, the results can be serious and devastating.

Retro-Virus and Humans

Science was not aware of such a deadly virus until a tragedy starting in the 1950s. In an attempt to inoculate people for polio, a vaccine was cultured by using the kidneys of monkeys in which the Retrovirus was present. This vaccine was administered directly into the blood stream of 98 million Americans who unknowingly received the Retrovirus called "Simian 40" or "Sim 40."

Retrovirus in humans can become active immediately or lay dormant for many years. It has been found dormant in regions of the nervous system for periods up to 30 years. It has been found hidden in areas of the lymphatic system and commonly appears in the blood. Little is known about what causes the Retrovirus to act up but we do know that it has a disastrous effect on the immune system and can reveal itself as the common cause of many diseases. It appears that this condition is more widespread than recognized. In this age the Retrovirus epidemic has claimed over one hundred and twenty-five million lives of men, women and children in Africa. This disaster is the result of a chicken-pox disease vaccine that has inflicted many with what they term "Slims Disease." In western countries, Retroviruses in combination with other viruses and fungi, cause several life-threatening afflictions.

HEPATITIS C (Non A or B)
ADULT T-CELL LEUKEMIA
HAIRY CELL LEUKEMIA
LYMPH CELL LEUKEMIA
FUNGAL LEUKEMIA
PERIPHERAL T-CELL LYMPHOMA
NON-HODGKINS LYMPHOMA
BREAST CANCER
LUPUS
MULTIPLE SCLEROSIS
BRAIN TUMORS

For years I went through all of the complications and frustrations from a Retrovirus laden Polio vaccine given to my youngest daughter. Those times were so difficult for her and fueled my search for a remedy. After many trials she is now healed. My discoveries and research are discussed in my booklet "RETROVIRUS THE NEW COMER." The treatment I have developed is called an X-40 kit. A unique kit that contains a tea mixture given to me by the American Indians. Combined with an herbal formula in capsules, a homeopathic liquid (90-22) and whole leaf, cold pressed aloe vera juice concentrate.

If the tumor is in the breast, also drain the breast in the following manner:

Breast Lumps

Breast lumps can be removed at an early stage, without surgery, by stimulating the lymph flow. Have the woman stand and have a second person, preferably the male energy of her husband, do the following: (for purposes of this example we will assume the lump is on the right side).

1   Stand on the right side of the standing patient. Put the spread fingers of the right hand on the right side of the sternum where the breast tissue attaches. Simultaneously put the spread fingers of the left hand on the right side of the spinal column, approximately parallel with the right hand. Hold for 60 seconds. Prayers for healing are entirely in order through these stages by both the subject and the practitioner.

2   While holding the left hand in the same place, move the right hand to a position directly in the arm pit, with the spread fingers extending straight down out of the arm pit. Again hold for 60 seconds.

3   Return to position one and hold for 60 seconds.

4   While holding the right hand in the same place on the right side of the sternum, shift the left hand to the position in the armpit and down from it. Hold for 60 seconds.

5   Return to position one and hold for 60 seconds.

6   Repeat this process 3 times a day until three days after the lump disappears. If the lump is on the left side, exchange the words right and left in the above instructions. If it does not disappear in three weeks, the case is more advanced and needs different care, including the possible use of magnets or fungus removing herbs. Of course, there is always the possibility the lump is something other than a blockage of the lymph glands.

Left   **Right**

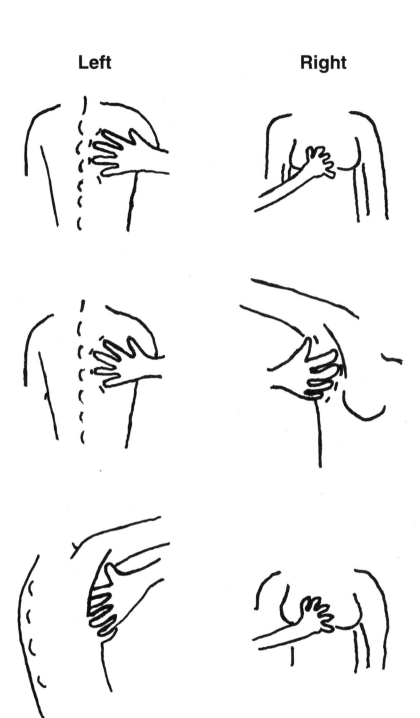

If the Retro-Virus tumor is in the brain, Tofu Compresses to the brain make a huge difference.

If the Retro-Virus tumor is in the male organs, make warm milk compresses.

To this type of cancer add to it as outlined in Concept No. II:
    zinc orotate
    calcium orotate
    magnesium orotate
and all the good things Concept II is offering.

New Concept No. III

Worms make tumors also

Worms often lump together and make tumors. They are mistaken for fungus tumors.

I have seen this very often, and Professor Brauchle in 1937 warned us to check for worm tumors.

Enclosed is a list of parasites.

> **ALL TYPES OF CANCER CASES**
> are afflicted with worms but
> they do not always make tumors.

To recognize Worm Tumors anywhere in the body, poke around the heels. If sore, watch out.

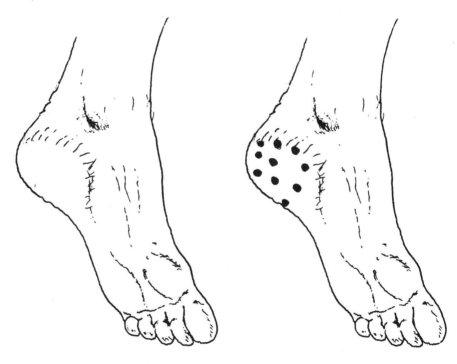

21

Removing Worms and Parasites
in the Management of Cancer

As I mentioned already, worms and parasites like a toxic medium, such as a toxic colon or toxic bodyfluid. Americans are the cleanest people. They shower or bathe every day. Daily a bunch of clothes goes into the washer, so it is *not* uncleanliness that makes worm eggs develop into destructive scavengers. It is the toxic medium caused by chemically affected food surroundings. The pH changes so much that even foreign scavengers such as bloodflukes and amoebas develop. All worms and parasites eat the best of the best of our body. All worms and parasites make the worst toxic waste, so they can multiply quickly and take over the host. All cancer patients have some form of worms, flukes, or parasites—that is the name of the game.

WORMS AND PARASITES

	Where found	Actions	What to do
AMOEBA	underdeveloped countries	attacks intestines liver eyes	go to physician, also homeopathic antidote
BLOOD FLUKES	underdeveloped countries parasites	attacks blood makes bloodclots strokes	see physician, also homeopathic antidote
FISH FLUKES	undercooked fish	cause skin trouble intestinal trouble	avoid all raw fish, homeopathic remedies
GIARDIA	unclean water	diarrhea intestinal trouble	see physician, also homeopathics

	Where found	Actions	What to do
HOOKWORM	horses, dogs and their feces	drinks up to 1/2 cup blood every day, anemia	see physician, also homeopathic remedy
INTESTINAL FLUKES	origin unknown	makes lots of mucous, sinus trouble	see physician, also homeopathic remedy
LIVER FLUKES	water plants growing in polluted water	simulates serious liver trouble	see physician, also homeopathic
LUNG FLUKES	origin unknown	shortness of breath, anemia	see physician, add homeopathic
PROTOZOA	wide spread in all countries	simulates arthritis leukemia Hodgkin's disease and many others	cuprium Ipecac Protozoa in homeopathic form
ROUND WORM	widespread in all countries	calcium deficiency children and adults	see physician, herbs for adults felix and cina for children
SALMONELLA	spoiled food also in chicken and some eggs	intestinal disorders, diarrhea, fever	apple cider vinegar
SPECIAL X	unknown	nervous system	Herb tea
TAPEWORM	the king of all worms	eats a lot and makes lots of toxins	see physician, also herbs

	Where found	Actions	What to do
THREADWORM	often found combined with Dioxin	anemia, itching all over	take homeopathic drops and see physician
TRICHINOSIS	pork and undercooked meat	attcks lungs, brain, heart, soft tissues	3 drops oil of wintergreen on 1 teaspoon molasses 2 times daily for 3 months
TOXOPLASMOSIS	cat feces	attacks fetus low bloodsugar	2 drops oil of sassafras 2 times daily to the sole of feet
WHIPWORM	origin unknown	combines with dioxin, nervous system	dioxin antidote with whipworm antidote

Lately, it was discovered, even announced on television, that a homoelytic parasite (blood parasite) was found in all cancer patients. It was so tiny, the announcer said, that many hundreds could live in a drop of blood. Very interesting, dear Channel 4 announcer. It is too bad you did not give us more help on the question, "What can we do about it?"

Calmirna figs have in their skins and kernels a substance which rips the skin of worms. It would be wise to eat some figs once in a while, just to make the environment in the intestine sweet and undesirable for the creature to live in.

See my book, "Parasites, The Enemy Within."

HERB FORMULAS

Dr. Rudolf Bruess of Austria, instructs his cancer patients to take the following juices, especially for fungus tumors:

Red beet juice	5 ounces
Carrot juice	12 ounces
Celery root juice	7 ounces
White radish juice	1/2 ounce

Celery juice is difficult to obtain. Biotta, a Swiss Company puts it out. Buy a case at a time.

Dr. Bruess also recommends potato peeling tea. Take unsprayed potatoes. Peel thickly. Boil 1 handful of peeling in 1 quart water for 20 minutes, strain. From this fluid take 3 tablespoons in 1 cup hot water and drink 3 cups a day. This cleans blood and lymphatic systems.

Cancer Formula from a Canadian Indian Princess

3 lbs. purple bergamot
3 lbs. burdock leaves
1 lb. and 1 oz. calamus root
1 lb. hops
12 ozs. wormwood
12 ozs. tansy

DIRECTIONS: Grind up, mix and take two 00-caps, three times a day or one teaspoon three times a day.

Formula for Bad Lungs: From a Minister

Garlic
Rosehip
Rosemary
Echinacea
Thyme (Spanish)

DIRECTIONS: Equal parts. Drink 3 cups of tea a day.

The famous Mr. Hoxey noticed his sick horses go to a certain spot in the meadow and eat only certain herbs. They went to this herb-rich patch of the meadow two times daily. The rest of the day they munched on grasses and whatever the farmer had to offer.

From this crude beginning, and through Mr. Hoxey's keen observation, the following terrific formula came on the market. You can buy the ingredients yourself or buy the ready-made pills.

Hoxey Formula

Red Clover Blossoms	Cascara Sagrada Bark
Chapparal	Sarsaparilla
Licorice Root	Prickly Ash Bark
Poke Root	Burdock Root
Peach Root	Buckthorn Bark
Oregon Grape Root	Norwegian Kelp
Stillingia	

DIRECTIONS: Begin by taking one capsule a day with a large glass of water, gradually increasing the dosage over a 2–3 week period one to two capsules three times daily.

Another Observation

A young farmer once came to me for help. A veterinarian had determined that his cow had a cancerous growth on her udder. I told him to take the cow out of the shed and lead the animal over the meadow, the garden, the hill and the riverside to see what kind of grasses and herbs the cow wanted. The farmer did what I told him to do and took his cow "out for dinner." She passed all the delicious herbs in the garden and the flowers and herbs on the meadow. Down near the river was a lonely cottonwood tree. The farmer took her there to rest and drink near the tree. Her tongue started lunging upwards and in and out of the mouth it went. She rubbed her shoulder on the tree trunk and mooed and licked and rubbed. The farmer climbed the tree and threw some branches to her. The cow became almost hysterical. Her appetite returned, and in less than two days, the cow was well. The farmer was overjoyed.

He asked me if his wife could drink this tea for the lumps in her breast. Since cottonwood leaves are not poisonous (the branches of the trees were used by the pioneers for women during childbirth), I saw no reason why his wife could not take it also. Sunday, after church, she confessed that all lumps were gone and they never came back.

**Scaly Red Skin Blemishes Which Do Not
Respond to Conventional Methods**

Take baking soda and moisten with camphor, make paste, apply overnight.
The late Dr. Carlton Frederichs taught us that skin cancer is related to T.B. Miasm.

Special Herbs in the additional management of Cancer

Lycopodium	If cancer is in liver 4 capsules a day.
Calamus root	If cancer is in lung. 1/2 teaspoon to a cup of water. 2 cups a day.
Nettle, Goldenrod	If cancer is in the kidney or if kidney shrinks.
2 parts of Calendula 1 part of Yarrow 1 part of Nettle	If cancer is in the colon. 1 quart a day.
Malva Vulgaris	If cancer is in the throat.

**Herbal Cancer Relief
Called Essiac**

6.5 cups dry Burdock Root cut
16 oz. weight Sheep Sorrel powdered
1 oz. weight Turkey Rhubarb Root powdered
4 oz. weight Slippery Elm Bark powdered
Mix ingredients
Use cast iron and/or stainless steel pots.
For all types of cancer.

Bring 2 gallons of mountain spring water to a boil. At sea level this takes about 30 minutes. Put essiac mixture in, let boil hard for 10 minutes. Turn off and let stand for 6 more hours. Turn on burner to high until it comes to a soft boil. This takes 20 minutes at sea level. Strain into 2nd pot with metal strainer, discard silt. Strain a 2nd time into first container. Funnel into bottles while warm. Use 16 oz. glass amber colored glasses. Refrigerate after opening. Store in a cool dry place when unopened. Take 4 tablespoons essiac with 4 tablespoons Mountain Spring Water on an empty stomach at bedtime.

Testimonials can be found in the book, "Calling Of An Angel" by Dr. Gary Glum. 5252 West Century Blvd. Suite 614, Los Angeles, CA 90045.

RELEASING POISONS IN THE MANAGEMENT OF CANCER

Hippocrates:

Diseases do not fall on us all of a sudden, diseases develop slowly by our daily sins against nature. After the accumulations of enough wrongdoings the body breaks down in disease.

Professor Dr. Katase, Osaha:

We have to fulfill a mission in regards to nutritional therapy. We have to secure the foundation of life of humanity now and for the coming season.

Professor Dr. Halden:

Comparatively few illnesses are of natural origin. Most illnesses are man-made.

Professor Dr. Kollath:

Lead is a protoplasmic poison, which means it interferes with the proper life-energy-enzyme exchange in the living body. It is amazing how beautifully our system is able to take this lead poison. Everyone has it, only a few people in very isolated places in the mountains or prairies are free from lead intoxications.

There is to be considered (1) the amount of lead in our system, and (2) the tolerance factor of lead and other metals such as arsenic, cadmium, mercury and copper. This tolerance factor differs in everyone. Some people sponge in more arsenic than others, some sponge in more lead, or aluminum-lead or mercury. I found that red-headed people are prone to take in more copper than others and orientals more mercury. The fair people sponge in more lead or lead aluminum, and men more cadmium than children or women. Also, the individual tolerance level differs widely. Children and adults under emotional stress have an affinity to arsenic. (See the excellent studies from Japan on "Leukemia—Emotions and Arsenic Poison.")

Chart of Metal Poisons

Name	Common Source	Effects/Symptoms	Suggested Help
Aluminum	Aluminum cookware, canned food and soda, foil, etc., antiacids, aluminum sulfate baking powders, toothpaste, soft water, and antiperspirants.	*Settles in* brain (neural tissue). *Symptoms include:* dryness of mouth, stomach pain, stomach ulcers, hard stool and/or with small hardened pieces ("fecal stones"), pain in spleen ares, forgetfulness, children cry a lot, kidney problem—esp. the right kidney, and cell oxidation inhibition. *Extreme toxicity leads to:* gastrointestinal irritation, colic, rickets, and convulsions.	*Protect with:* Vitamin E, C, Metaline. *Help with:* Aluminae 6x-12x, or Co Enzyme International.
Arsenic	Household and garden pesticides, insecticides via chemical called arsenoxide (both use and manufacture process). Coal burning, tobacco smoke, defoliants, metal smelting, manufacturing of glass, dental compounds for root canal fillings.	*Settles in* the muscles and the brain (dislodging phosphorus). *Symptoms include:* sweet metallic taste, garlicky odor to breath and stool, constriction of throat, difficulties in swallowing, burning sensation (inflammation) in eyes, throat and chest, enlargement of tonsils, muscle spasms, pain in muscles of the back, adjustments to spine do not "hold." *Extreme toxicity leads to:* mild gastrointestinal disturbances, anorexia, low	*Protect with:* Iodine, selenium, sulfur bath, amino acids, Vitamin C. *Help with:* Arsenicum 6x, or Harpagophytum tea, or Tea with equal portions of grassia, white oak bark, and golden rod. Drink 2 cups daily.

Name	Common Source	Effects/Symptoms	Suggested Help
Arsenic continued		grade fever with changes in white blood count, weakness (fatigue, listlessness, low vitality), brittle nails, loss of hair, skin color changes, dark spots, localized edema, and nervousness. *Since arsenic has a constricting effect on the muscle structure, and loves to lodge in muscles, **the most outstanding symptom is the constant backache.***	
Cadmium	Industrial exposure (e.g., from activities involving electroplating, low melting alloys, solders, batteries, pigments, barrier in atomic fission control, etc.), dental partial dentures, tobacco leaves, tobacco smoke, welding, paints, oxide dusts, contaminated drinking water, galvanized pipes, pigments, contaminated shellfish from industrial seashores.	*Settles in* heart and right kidney, and effects proper functioning of several enzymes. *Symptoms include:* Pneumonitis, vomiting diarrhea, loss of calcium in bones, deterioration of heart and blood vessel structures, and prostration. *Extreme toxicity leads to:* Hypertension, kidney damage, loss of sense of smell (anosmia), emphysema, and decreased appetite.	*Protect with:* Zinc, calcium, sulfur bath, amino acids, paprika, Vitamin C. *Help with:* Cadmium-X 12x-30x
Copper	Copper pipes and cooking utensils.	*Settles in* brain and ovaries. *Symptoms include:* Burning sensation in throat and tonsils.	*Help with:* Cuprum, or Zinc with B6

Name	Common Source	Effects/Symptoms	Suggested Help
Copper continued		*Extreme toxicity* *leads to:* Wants to open hands all the time.	
Gold		*Extreme toxicity* *leads to:* Tingling through system.	*Help with:* Aurum
Graphite	Pencils, tires, lubricants.	*Settles in* heart. *Extreme toxicity* *leads to:* Sense of numbness all over body.	*Help with:* Graphite (homeopathic), or Breathe in steam of poppyseeds, and drink poppyseed tea.
Lead	Paints, water pipes, tin cans, insecticides, motor vehicle exhaust (leaded gas), tobacco smoke, "moonshine" whiskey, newsprint & colored ads, hair dyes and rinses, dolomite, soft coal, leaded glass, pewter ware, pesticides, pencils, fertilizers, pottery, cosmetics, tobacco smoke, polluted air. Is a *protoplasmic poison* found in bleached white sugar.	*Settles into* liver, kidneys, spleen, and bone marrow. *Symptoms include:* abdominal pain, anemia, enzyme poisoning, lowered osteoblast (bone) production, lowered blood formation, blockage of enzymes at cellular level, and lesions of the central and peripheral nervous system. *The central nervous system lesions result in behavioral problems such as hyperactivity in children.* *Extreme toxicity* *leads to:* weakness, listlessness, fatigue, pallor, abdominal discomfort, constipation, hyperactive children, mad and weakened condition, lack of will power, lack of abstract thinking, lack of	*Protect with:* Sulfur bath, amino acids, Vitamin C, E, calcium iron. *Help with:* Plumbum, or Boil 3 teasp. whole cloves in 1 qt. cranberry juice for 20 min. Stir and add 3 qt. more juice. Now add 1 tsp. cream of tartar. Stir. Drink 5 oz. 3x daily. For children 3 oz. 3x daily for 12–15 days. Then do it once a week, or make Tea using using mixture of: 6 oz. basil, 1 oz. rosemary, 1 oz. hyssop, 1 oz. boneset. Drink 1 cup 3x daily, or make Tea using mixture of: Cloves and Vitamin C, or Red Cabbage, or Chamomile tea (to rebuild calcium after removing lead).

Name	Common Source	Effects/Symptoms	Suggested Help
Lead continued		mental capacity, tooth decay, allergic reactions to food and environment, increases in diabetes and multiple sclerosis. **Lead is a proto-plasmic poison, which means it interferes with the proper life-energy-enzyme exchange in the living body.**	
Mercury	Manufacture and delivery of petroleum products, fungicides (for grains and cereals), fluorescent lamps, cosmetics, hair dyes, barometers, thermometers, amalgams in dentistry, salt water fish caught in con-taminated waters, medications (diuretics).	*Settles in* liver, spleen, kidneys, intestinal wall, heart, skeletal muscles, lungs, and bones. *Symptoms include:* Loss of appetite and weight, severe emo-tional disturbances, tremors, blood changes, inflammation of gums, chewing and swallowing difficulty, loss of sense of pain. Cell destruction, blocked transport of sugars (energy at cell level), increased per-meability of potassi-um, convulsions, irregular heart beat, kidney, malfunction. *Extreme toxicity leads to:* excessive salivation, metallic taste, blue line develops along the gingival margin, gums become hyper-trophied, bleed easily and are sore, and teeth become loose.	*Protect with:* Pectin, sulfur bath, amino acids, Vitamin C, selenium. *Help with:* Mercurium, or Green algae

Name	Common Source	Effects/Symptoms	Suggested Help
Mercury continued		Tremors of the eyelids, lips, tongue, fingers and extremities. Coarse jerky movements and gross incoordination interfere with fine movements such as writing and eating. Visual deterioration, and dysphagia (difficulty in speaking). Atrophy of the cerebellar cortex, and to a lesser extent the cerebral cortex occurs. Microscopic changes occur in the granular layer of the cerebellum, ganglion cells, and posterior columns.	
Nickel	Used to make hardened fats. Commonly found in all margarines, as well as oils and fats labeled **hydrogenated,** meaning hardened vegetable oil. *Be sure to check labels* of all prepared foods for use of **hydrogenated** or **partially hydrogenated** oils, including breads, chips, cookies, candies, etc.	*Settles in* sinus, joints, and spinal column. *Symptoms include:* backache, headache, stuffed up sinuses, listlessness, swollen joints (knee, wrist, and ankle), and painful cracking neck. *Extreme toxicity leads to:* paralysis, overflow of blood to brain, and epilepsy.	*Protect with:* 1 tbs. of poppyseeds with honey by mouth 2x daily, poppyseed cake. *Help with:* Nickel (homeopathic), or Breathe in steam of poppyseeds, and drink poppyseed tea, or Apply poppyseed compress to affected area of body.
Silver	Photography, dental fillings.	*Extreme toxicity leads to:* Cold numbness through heart region, heavy weight on hands and feet.	*Help with:* Argentum
Tin		*Extreme toxicity leads to:* Cold, icy feeling throughout body, numbness of feet.	*Help with:* Stannum

Universal Remedies To Remove Metal Poisons

1. Mix 2 tbs. pumpkin seeds (ground) and 1 tbs. okra powder. Add 1/2 tsp. cayenne pepper. Take 1 tsp. of mixture with about 1 tbs. of rhubarb sauce, 3x daily for 10 days. *(Most effective with lead, arsenic, platinum, gold, and mercury.)*

2. Eat zucchini and green beans exclusively for three days.

3. Eat squash and strawberries. *(Most effective for arsenic poison, especially good for smokers.)*

4. Boil 3 teasp. of green beans in water until done. Add 2 lbs. finely chopped celery and 4 lbs. coarsely cut zucchini. Boil another 5 min. or until zucchini is done. Remove from fire and add 3 bunches of finely chopped parsley. Season with spice. Eat only this for three days, make more if finished before three days. When reheating take only a portion from the refrigerator. Eat as often as you want. Drink parsley tea or willow leaf tea as a beverage. *(Most effective in removing metals lodged in glands and nerves.)*

5. METALINE: an herbal remedy composed of pumpkin seed, okra, rhubarb root, cayenne pepper, and dulse.

6. Sulfur baths in natural springs or via granules, tablets or powders added to the bath water. *(Most effective for lead, arsenic, platinum, gold, and mercury.)*

7. Add 7 oz. liquid Clorox to warm bath in good sized bathtub. Bathe 10–15 min. *Note: not everyone can take Clorox baths, so check by soaking feet in a weak solution (1 tsp. to one gallon of water).*

8. Make a mixture of 4 oz. cranberry juice and 4 oz. distilled water. Take mixture 4x daily for 3 days, then wait 5 days and repeat.

HERBICIDE

Herbicide contains Dioxin. Dioxin is Agent Orange. This broadleaf defoliant was used in Vietnam. It is used, so our lawns will not have dandelions or other broadleaved healing plants.

All poisons make a medium in which parasites, flukes and worms thrive. Dioxin however takes the cake. It binds these scavengers so tightly that ordinary antiparasitic measures do not work. You have to have Dioxin Antidote with it.

MINERALS IN THE
MANAGEMENT OF CANCER

Professor Dr. W. Haupke:
Fifteen years ago, trace minerals were almost unknown. Nowadays, our knowledge is profound enough to realize that trace minerals are vital for the human body. We know that certain illnesses develop out of lack of trace minerals.

Hippocrates:
Illnesses do not come over us from somewhere and all of a sudden. They develop slowly from our "daily wrongs" against nature. When there are enough "wrongs" built up, they appear all at once and suddenly.

Dr. Kuhl, M.D.
Vitamin and mineral deficiencies can lead to tumor and cancer formation.

CHLORIDE

Chloride is a component of hydrochloric acid. It maintains the acid/base balance. There is a link between chlorinated water and cancer of the gastrointestinal and urinary tract, so supplements not recommended in the treatment of cancer or candida! Refined salt like Morton's is full of chloride not balanced with other minerals like sea salt! Eat sea salt only!

GERMANIUM

Dr. Levine said that germanium "activates or substitutes for oxygen." Dr. Asai discussed its chelating effects on heavy metals like cadmium. Germanium seems to have a cancer pain relieving effect.

The little district of Daun, West Germany, is rested peacefully and quietly in the setting of the old Vulcanic Mountains of the Eifel.

The lush green meadows, the wind swept trees, the little farms, and the quaint villages do not look different than they do in other parts of the country, and yet, the Daun District is entering the limelight of the world.

In 1944, several researchers became aware of the fact that in Daun, there was no cancer to speak of. A district without cancer. And those that had cancer when they came there were healed when they lived there for six months or longer.

At first, the scientists examined the soil and plants of this area. Finally, they found that the water of this area was different. It contained more Magnesium Chloride than other waters. They found 0.45659 mg. magnesium chloride per liter

37

of water. Magnesium Chloride is an activator of many, many enzymes. It is also needed in the breakdown of protein to Amino Acids, the building stones of the body. Magnesium Chloride is also known to activate the Ester complexes. Much later, it was found that it was not the magnesium, but another element. It was *germanium* which was unique as a trace mineral in the waters of the Daun. This water is distributed as Dunaris Healing Water. Researchers went on the hot line to find out all they could about germanium.

Germanium is used in the electro-magnetic industry to guide and focus energies. "Wild energies" become tamed with germanium. When I place my hand on a growth, I feel energies boiling, dashing, whirling, rushing, without guidance in an unbelievable turmoil. Of all the nations, Japan is far ahead with her research on germanium and cancer. North Korea has a district (like Daun) where hardly any cancer is found. This area has a very high content of germanium in the water and plants. Ginseng from Korea has the ability to accumulate more germanium than any other plant, and therefore, is greatly appreciated for its healthful benefits.

Sick Koreans go to the woods and search for a lichen which they eat. They also place lichens on tumors to reduce the size and pain. This lichen is loaded with germanium.

Here in America, we have good sources of germanium also. We have a spring which has the same mineral content as Dunaris Healing Water. We have clays (in Wyoming) and best of all we have corn. The Blue Corn (Squaw Corn) and the Indian Corn (Colored Kernels) are the richest of all the corn varieties for minerals and trace minerals, including germanium. A scientist from Rocky Flats was in such bad shape that death seemed just a few steps away. I asked him which foods he really liked. After a long while, he said, "the morning mush made out of corn is the only thing I can eat." So, I told him to eat blue corn mush, mornings, noon and night or whenever he felt like it. Two weeks later, he had discarded all food supplements, but ate mush, corn grits and mush again. A few weeks later he was strong and now, after years, is working full blast.

Germanium in a natural state is in sprouted alfalfa and other sprouts. It is also available in tablet form.

POTASSIUM

Potassium maintains osmotic pressure inside cells. It activates cellular respiration as it is a catalyst in the release of energy, protein and glycogen synthesis. LOSS OCCURS IN CATABOLISM? Magnesium deficiency depletes potassium. It also helps maintain acid/base balance. This is highly recommended in cancer treatment. *Mix capsules or crush pills in water to take because they can burn your stomach lining. It is better to take frequent smaller doses than one large dose.*

SODIUM

Sodium maintains osmotic pressure outside cells. It inhibits cellular respiration and washes out potassium in the amounts found in the American diet. It is part of the digestive juices and thus counteracts excess acidity. Use sea salt for a healthier balance of minerals.

SELENIUM

Still not enough studies have been made on Selenium, the "new trace mineral" with lots of potential. Up to now we know that selenium is needed to:

1. fight infection
2. detoxify many common pollutants
3. protect the heart, especially when combined with vitamin E
4. make beautiful skin and give good vision

It also has something to do with cancer treatment. It is not understood how selenium accomplishes all that and more research has to follow. In all cases given, it uplifts the outlook on life. The sadness, despair and melancholy which is often seen in cancer victims is miraculously lifted. These people can take a hold of themselves again. Selenium promotes deeper sleep. Selenium gives a restful mind and peace within.

Selenium joins with glutathione to become cathione peroxidase and destroys dangerous peroxides free radicals. Do not use too much selenium, take it only from natural sources.

The main supplies are fish and liver. Dr. Gerson gave his patients lots of liver to eat. Nowadays liver is only safe when the animal has had no stilbesterol in the feed. I am more inclined to eat seafood. Mushrooms, good eggs, onion, and garlic are rich in selenium. Wheat and wheat products (if the wheat is organically grown) are also good sources of selenium.

Dr. Gertard Schrauzer, Prof. of Chemistry at the University of California at San Diego, said: "Selenium is one of the most efficient agents in stimulating the natural defense system against cancer."

SULPHUR

Sulphur, magnesium, and germanium are the stars of the cancer diet. They play a major role in B vitamin co-enzymes and in deactivating free radicals. Many hundreds of liver enzymes contain sulphur as it is integrated into the structure of your entire body. It is a component of mucus and is indispensable to immune function. Sulphurasis, cruciferous vegetables such as cabbage, broccoli, cauliflower, etc., are being heavily promoted by the American Cancer Society as an adjunct to conventional treatment and preventative measure.

ZINC

Chronic diseases are characterized by long-term mineral deficiencies, with zinc deficiencies being most commonly found.

Why is zinc necessary?

Fifty-nine or more enzymes require zinc for their functions or as part of their structure. Zinc is essential in the elimination of carbon dioxide in cellular respiration. It is involved in RNA and DNA synthesis and the incorporation of methionine into protein. It helps protect fats from oxidation and mobilizes Vitamin A from the liver. It assists in hormone metabolism. Zinc is needed for all wound healing— whether from trauma or surgery. It is also important for the proper function of the pancreas (insulin production), thyroid, thymus and the immune system. Zinc also counteracts heavy-metal poisons (lead, cadmium and others) and helps prostate function and the reproductive organs. It helps too in managing multiple sclerosis, in overcoming skin problems and for the prevention of cataracts.

Why are we so in need of zinc when plants have it? Reason: plants grown with chemical fertilizer and other chemicals are not producing the link to zinc absorption by the cells of the body, and that link need is *picolinic acid*. Picolinic acid has nothing to do with pickles or cucumbers; it is an enzyme-hormone. Without this the human body cannot utilize zinc. And that is "the missing link," ZINC PICOLINATE.

Remember, the earmark of chronic diseases is mineral and trace mineral deficiencies caused by zinc malabsorption. ZINC PICOLINATE is a breakthrough in nutrition as nothing before. Let's overcome chronic diseases!

The National Cancer Institute reported zinc along with magnesium as two factors that inhibit carcinogenesis. Liver and sunflower seeds are rich in zinc. Small frequent doses are recommended.

VITAMINS IN THE MANAGEMENT
OF ALL TYPES OF CANCER

Dr. Kuhl, M.D.:
Vitamin and mineral deficiencies can lead to tumor and cancer formation.

Dr. Kollath, M.D.:
Cancer is the end result of years of poor nutrition and an unhealthy life style.

VITAMIN A

Two cancer researchers from the National Cancer Institute's 1974 symposium report that they were able to prevent cancer in the windpipe of laboratory animals by giving them supervised amounts of Vitamin A. Furthermore, scientists report that the vitamin can even help reverse cancer proliferation, if the patient is treated early enough in the illness.

> *NOTE: "This offers hope for a natural source for protection and/or reversal of cancer, an increasingly common fatal ailment,"* said Thomas Maugh, Ph.D.

More Discoveries Announced. As reported in *Science* magazine (December 1974), other researchers have found that Vitamin A has a definite anti-cancer role. Thomas H. Maugh, Ph.D., suggests that cells may be protected after exposure to cancer by the action of Vitamin A. It is believed, says Dr. Maugh, that the vitamin helps to "medicate a return to normalcy" after the damage has taken place, and this protects against more full-blown "transformation" of the cell to malignancy at a later date.

Dr. Maugh:
Vitamin A alerts the body's own built-in defenses to help reverse the cell damage caused by the carcinogen and therefore prevent the cell's eventual surrender to cancer. Furthermore, Vitamin A helps the body's defense system destroy cancerous cells.

B_{15}

The whole vitamin B complex group is needed to sustain good health. Nature intended to create all B vitamins in the small intestine but our mode of living does not justify the assumption any longer that all of us have sufficient B vitamins. We don't have to go to pills, we can take Rice polishings (women) or brewers yeast (men). But for many it becomes easier to swallow a pill than to stir, mix, splash, and make faces.

41

There are two outstanding vitamins which are rarely discussed: B_{15} and B_{17}. B_{15}, also called pangamic acid, is a special one. It brings more oxygen to the tissue. It opens up the veins, arteries and capillaries so more oxygen supply can be furnished to the cells. Vitamin E also is an oxygen supplier and oxygen saver, but it does it only for the inner organs such as the liver, pancreas, heart and lungs. The two are a perfect couple. In Russia B_{15}, A, and E are routinely given to people over 50 and for all kinds of illnesses. Since in most illnesses we deal with a lack of oxygen supply, this knowledge becomes tremendously handy. *See findings of Dr. Otto Warburg.*

B_{17}

B_{17} is not a newcomer. It has been used for a long time. Researchers found B_{17} in over one thousand plants. In bitter almonds and apricot kernels; it is present in the most concentrated form, but millet and all seeds show B_{17} in appreciable amounts.

The Chinese used bitter almond tea for tumors as far back as 3,500 years ago. It has been used in the Eastern World for centuries as: an extract, a tea, and an infusion. In Turkey apricot kernels are combined with figs and eaten as a special treat for Cancer-sick folks.

The Greeks and Romans used bitter almond water medicinally and called it Amygdalarum amarum. As early as 1845, Fedor Inosemzov, the Russian physician, combined bitter and sweet almonds for two kinds of "fungus-like tumors."

In the year 1830, the chemist, Robiquot and Boutron isolated B_{17} also called Amygdalin in its pure form. Only seven years later in 1837, the Scientists Liebig and Woehler discovered that Amygdalin is split by an enzyme complex into:

1 Molecule of Hydrogen Cyanide
1 Molecule of Benzaldehyde
2 Molecules of Sugar

GUIDE TO B_{17} FOODS

Kernels or seeds of fruits. The highest concentration of Vitamin B_{17} is found in nature in the form of bitter almonds, apples, apricots, cherries, nectarines, peaches, pears, plums, and prunes.

Beans: broad (Vicia faba), burma, chick peas, lentils (sprouted), lima, mung (sprouted), Rangoon, scarlet runner.

Nuts: bitter almond, macadamia.

Berries: (almost all wild berries): blackberry, chokeberry, Christmas berry, cranberry, elderberry, raspberry, strawberry.

Seeds: chia, flax, sesame, clover.

Grains: oat groats, barley, brown rice, buckwheat groats, chia, flax, millet, rye, and wheat berries.

In the Himalayan Mountains of Pakistan lives an isolated tribe of people. They live in a beautiful valley called the Hunzaland. Travelers reported that the Hunzakuts are very healthy. Their women at the age of eighty look as we do at forty years of age. This sparked the interest of physicians such as Dr. Allen E. Banik, an optometrist, who was accompanied by some of his companions. They travelled the lengthy and dangerous roads on foot and horse, and found what was reported to be true. These peoples' diet consisted of lots of apricots, vegetables, millet and other grains. After Dr. Banik and Renee Taylor published their book on the Hunzaland we all started eating dried apricots.

The next explorers also found that they cracked the seeds of the apricots, so we started to eat the seeds to keep our figures and health at age 40. However, nothing spectacular happened. Then I read a book from a nature lover who reported the fabulous scenery, with the gushing waters coming down from the high mountains which were white with minerals rushing through the entire territory of the Hunzaland. It was reported that the inhabitants treat this water like a holy spring. No garbage is thrown into it. They use the water only for their gardens and for their water supply in the houses. This pure water is loaded with calcium carbonate. Here lies the secret of the Hunzakuts' fabulous health.

> Apricots provide enzymes
> Apricot kernels have B_{17}, the longevity factor of the cells. Calcium Carbonate, or lime water, is needed to make the enzymes in the apricot active so that this enzyme can assimilate vitamin B_{17}.

Whether B_{17} cures Cancer or not is not for me to say, but it surely takes pain away. B_{17} brightens the dark days of a Cancer Victim. Patients are feeling better and happier. All cases are eating better, gaining weight, and strength.

Dr. Dean Burk, head of the Cytochemistry Section of the National Cancer Institute, Bethesda, Maryland, said "B_{17} is non-toxic." After testing B_{17} on rats he said, "Aspirin tablets proved to be twenty times more toxic to the animals than Amygdalin."

Here is your homemade B_{17}:

> 4 apricot kernels
> 2 pieces dried apricots
> 5 calcera carb., 6x homeopathic, or limewater

Chew this. Take the formula twice a day. It tastes wonderful. Everybody should have this treat, at least once a day!

Commercially, B_{17} is called laetrile. There are two kinds of laetrile: one is female in nature and one is male in nature. Therefore sometimes it helps and sometimes it doesn't. The controversy is on. The natural product as indicated has both male and female aspects and the body picks what is needed.

43

NUTRITION IN THE MANAGEMENT
OF ALL TYPES OF CANCER

According to the world famous cancer research physician, Dr. Hans Nieper of Germany: "In Germany it is a law. When someone has cancer, doctors must tell the patient that there are four alternatives:

surgery
radiation
chemotherapy or
nutrition

The doctor must explain nutrition to the patient, and the patient may take the choice."

What is "Correct Nutrition"

Many books have been written on this subject. In essence they contain the following:

1) quality of food
2) quantity of food
3) proper preparation of food
4) electro-magnetic energy in food
5) food combining

Quality of Food

The industrial treatments of natural foods has in no way increased the *quality of food*. The accumulative effects of chemicals, additives, and colorings are discussed at length in many pamphlets and books. The advantage of long shelf-life of cereals, flours, ready-made products, oils, fats, breads and other necessities of life carry a stigma of dark angels with them. The dark angels bring suffering and ruination of good health.

The terrible human suffering of added hormones to the feed of animals is rarely discussed. Chicken, eggs, milk and meat still carry the hormonal additives that can make large changes in the male-female relationship of humans. The delicate hormone balance is constantly upset. The very cell is in an uproar. Here are some experts speaking:

Dr. Kotshan (MD):

"Our civilization thinks and teaches that by beautifying natural foods, its quality could be improved. However, applying our advanced technology to food preparation, preservation, packaging and manhandling, the biological substance of our entire population is at stake."

Dr. Kollath (MD):

"The nutritional crisis in which we are now is something new in history. The change in the quality of food by taking natural substances away and replacing them with artificial additives will always denature the food value and serious consequences have to be expected."

Dr. Vollati also said:

"Denatured nutrition can destroy the best nation and, therefore, it should be in the interest of the government to protect its subjects from using denatured food."

The Preparation of Foods

The *preparation of food* starts with shopping. Farmers Markets are the best. Here one can find a great selection of home-grown vegetables, delicious unsprayed apples, tree-ripened fruit, and berries of all kinds. The pure honey and fertile eggs!!! The chickens run and have exercise. They are fed grains and greens so you can taste the goodness of nature in every egg. But most of us have to go to Super Markets. The fruit was picked green for transportation's sake, particularly the tomatoes, which are usually tasteless. The colored oranges and the waxed cucumbers look beautiful. There again, we find industrialization for beauty's sake.

We know the dangers of pesticides, coloring, additives, and preservatives. We know that all these things have an accumulative, detrimental effect on the body's reserves. Alkaline Acid imbalance becomes a contributing factor to severe illnesses when enough poisons enter the tissues.

There are several proven methods to counteract the foreign substances in food, vegetables, milk, water, fruit and everything else consumed.

Linda Clark speaks on detoxifying fruit and vegetables by placing them in a very light solution of Chlorox.

> One teaspoon Chlorox to one gallon water
> Place vegetables or fruit in solution and soak for ten minutes.
> Rinse carefully. Store in refrigerator until use.

However, many of us are allergic to Chlorox, and liquids can not be detoxified this way.

For many years the "Soma board" has been on the market. This has kept many, many families in excellent health. It is made with herbs, crystals, magnetic alloids, and other items. It lasts for 16 years. Just place foods, milk and juices on or around it.

Detoxifying is a process of neutralizing chemicals and additives in food or liquids so they become harmless to the body. Detoxifying foods will not improve the mineral or vitamin content of such treated foods. Mineral deficient merchandise will stay that way; however, the small amount of minerals present can be assimilated completely.

The Body is an Electro-Chemical Energy System

This energy system needs fuel to function properly. It needs fuel that has energy to give. Foods that have been manhandled—canned and filled with additives, irradiated, microwaved and wrongly combined—will not release sufficient energies to keep us going. Nor will it keep our brain at high gear or keep us free from disease. "Disruption of cellular energy is what we label disease." I heard this sentence stated by a medical doctor and it hit me—this is heavenly truth!

Scientists tell us that the amount of food and fluid we take in is eliminated at the same ratio as ingested, ounce by ounce and pint by pint. What we live on is the electro-chemical energy created—emanated from our food and fluids. If we continue to take in food which is low in electro-chemical power we lower our resistance. This means that we cannot ward off environmental poisons which are in water, air and food.

Today, we have to create a different way of eating and adapt a different lifestyle. Understanding kitchen chemistry is a must in order to keep our family alive and healthy. Dr. Parcels said: "The relation of foods one to another will greatly establish the electro-chemical energies." She also said, "these energies need a slightly acid environment to function." If the environment is too *alkaline*, the *functions* of electro-chemical energies will slow down or stop entirely depending on the amount of alkalinity.

Electro-chemical energies are destroyed in over-cooked foods, old food, over ripe food, irradiated food and food that passed through a scanning machine in stores. The most important cause, however, is our habit of wrong food combination.

How to Combine Foods for Best Electro-Chemical Energy

> Bread and cheese is a no-no.
> Bread and meat is a no-no.
> Bread and chicken is a no-no.
> Macaroni and cheese is a no-no.

Citrus fruit and grains make a tough mucus in the stomach and in the sinuses; other fruits and grains will not do that. Sweet fruit is a desirable food but must be eaten as a meal or between meals. Only the apple is neutral and can be eaten with vegetables or meats. Apple sauce and stewed apples are fine.

47

DO NOT EAT FRUIT AND VEGETABLES TOGETHER.

MEAT AND MILK IS A NO-NO.

Meats need vinegar used as a salad dressing (acids) to be prepared for digestion. If you drink milk with meats, the hydrochloric acid (HCL) is neutralized and the meat rots in the stomach.

Grains and meats are a very poor combination, so are grains and cheeses. Think of your sandwich at noon! You become tired and listless after a double decker!

Fruits are fine mixed, cut in cubes or whole, but do not eat nuts with it. If you put nuts with your fruit salad, your fruit salad has no vibration.

Carrots and peas mixed look so pretty and so inviting but it will not feed your body through the electro-chemical function. It becomes a ballast.

THE APPLE IS THE EXCEPTION!
RICE IS AN EXCEPTION!

Apples in all forms can be mixed with vegetables. Rice can be taken with protein.

The Electro-Chemical diet makes your life light burn brightly. Where there is light, the darkness has to disappear. The atomic influences, the chemicalization, and the metallic poison cannot easily disturb the balance in you. It is the way of survival.

A good dinner consisting of salad, vegetables, meat or chicken, and/or cheese, should never have a dinner roll with it. A dinner roll by itself may serve as a snack between meals or before bedtime. If you are in need of putting on weight, have a roll before bedtime with plenty of butter!

This researcher is very well known and his findings are well founded. The result is excellent. He improves cell respiration by taking cold pressed oils in salads, cottage cheese and in vegetables. He gives yoghurt, sauerkraut, cottage cheese, kefir, buttermilk, fermented vegetable juices, and in particular fermented beet juice. Vegetables and fruits should be organically grown, i.e., without spray or artificial fertilizers. Carbohydrates and sugar are not on the menu. Some eggs and fowl are permitted.

When you first get out of bed in the morning:
   Drink diluted cherry juice
   or lemon juice and water
   or cranberry with lemon peel, soaked overnight.
Breakfast:
   fruit and flax seed ground up
   or, barley with honey, cream and fruit
   or, millet cereal with cream and cottage cheese with oil
   or, a slice of whole wheat bread
Juice for in-between meals. Beet or carrot juice.
Lunch:
   Have cooked vegetables, a raw vegetable salad, and
   fish, or chicken, or lamb.
Afternoon:
   Fruit and whole wheat toast if desired.
Supper:
   Have raw salad, rice, asparagus, yoghurt, vegetables. No animal protein at night.

The reason for not having protein at night is: If you eat protein such as chicken, eggs, fish or meats, it takes the body 8 hours to break the protein down to amino acids. The building stones of the tissue is Amino Acid. The carrier of these valuable amino acids is the lymph system. At night the lymph system closes down to low function, and the liver will dump the building stones into the cancer growth. When you eat protein at night you feed your cancer but starve your body.

SPECIAL FORMULAS IN THE MANAGEMENT OF CANCER

HIGH MINERAL BROTH

Wash well and peel 2 quarts potatoes. Discard potatoes and use peel only.
To each cup potato peels add 2 cups of water.
Simmer 1 hour or until very soft. Mash well, drain off liquid.
Drink 4 oz. of liquid morning, and 4 oz. at noon.

BLOOD AND TISSUE CLEANSING PLAN

Start this diet plan with this thorough cleansing plan. Repeat cleansing plan
one day every other month.
Morning: 1 quart unsweetened grape juice
Noon: 1 quart orange juice (canned or fresh)
        2 thick slices *raw* onion
3 P.M. 1 quart pineapple or prune juice
Evening: 1 quart grapefruit or orange juice (canned or fresh)
        2 thick slices *raw* onion

BLOOD FEEDING

Clean well large turnips (rutabagas or yellow turnips when in season).
Dice into 1 inch pieces. Cover with distilled water. Simmer until soft.
Mash liquid in well and strain through very fine screen or cheese cloth.
Drink 1 quart of this liquid every day.
    Under sterilized sanitation, this has been scientifically proven. The above for-
mula if given intravenously—works like a miracle—used instead of blood trans-
fusion—it never fails.

CALCIUM NORMALIZING BROTH

1 teacup unprocessed bran. (consult your health food store.) Add
1 quart distilled water.
Bring to a boil over low flame, remove at once and let stand for 2 hours.
Strain as you use. Sweeten with honey. Drink 8 oz. twice daily.

DIGESTIVE SYSTEM NORMALIZER

Chop, grate or slice thin, 1 quart white or red cabbage. Add 1 quart water. Boil 1/2 hour or until soft. Draw off liquid. Use 4 oz. of liquid each day. Supplies vitamin U, Alkalime, sulphur, calcium, zinc, phosphorus, iron, copper, vitamin C, A, B_1, G.

Here are some hints on how to protect yourself against poisons.
—Drink catnip tea for arsenic poisoning.
—Drink mandrake root tea after you've taken poisoned water.
—Drink pokeberry tea for sodium fluoride poison.
—Put green grass in a bottle. Let it stand for two hours—This also binds sodium fluoride to the green.
—For fallout take a soda and salt bath.

The following recipe removes lead from your tissue:

1 gallon cranberry juice
2 tbsp. whole cloves
2 tsp. ground cinnamon
1 tsp. cream of tartar

DIRECTIONS: Boil the cloves in 1 quart cranberry juice for 20 minutes. Strain and add two tsp. ground cinnamon. Stir and add it to the rest of the cranberry juice. Now add 1 tsp. cream of tartar. Stir. Drink 5 ounces 3 times daily. For children, 3 ounces 3 times daily for 12–15 days. Then do it once a week.

LEUKEMIA

Leukemia does not make tumors, so it does not belong to the tumor making diseases. It causes swelling of the Lymph glands.

LEUKEMIA AND ITS MANAGEMENT

I had the good fortune to be working as a registered nurse in Dresden, Germany, at a 2000 bed hospital for natural healing which was headed by Dr. Brauchle. There he stated the following truth on leukemia: "Leukemia is not cancer of the blood." He taught that there are 3 causes of leukemia:

No. 1   The disintegration of the blood is caused by a malfunctioning of the Portal Vein System. The Portal Vein System is the system that draws the nourishment out of the food we eat and also converts Prana into life energy.

No. 2   Most leukemic cases are found in homes where husband and wife fight. Or in cases of divorce, or when the spiritual need of a child or an adult is not understood.
In short, it is a love situation. The Portal Vein system is extremely sensitive to emotions and will close shut if something is wrong emotionally. Please have a happy table surrounding when you eat. No fighting, no shout outs, no ugly words. The poisons so created is a cause for the digestion to close down the Portal Vein's functioning.

No. 3   Most all leukemic patients have a tailbone displacement. Go to a chiropractor and have the tailbone put back in order. The tailbone is the pump for the spinal fluid. If the pump is stuck, the spinal fluid and also the cerebral fluid will not function. The tailbone also is taking care of the waste product of the nervous system.

IMPORTANT

Repeated nosebleed in children should always be treated by a physician. One to two years before a "blood break down," a period of nosebleeds is experienced.

This is what we did in Professor Brauchle's hospital of Natural Healing:

First the tailbone had to be set.

Nurses had to prepare and give the following delicious drink to all leukemia cases. Besides the main kitchen in the huge establishment, there was a diet kitchen on each floor. We loved those diet kitchens. They were large, handsome, and light, while the pharmacy department next door was small, compact, and had only a small window. In the kitchen we prepared:

1 pint white grapefruit juice
1 pint freshly squeezed orange juice
1 pint grape juice
1 pint water with the juice of three limes
1 pint water with the juice of two lemons
1 pint frozen pineapple juice diluted
1 pint papaya juice, diluted

Take 12 whole eggs and 6 egg yolks. Beat eggs very thoroughly and mix into fruit juice mixture. Sweeten with honey if needed. For a change of taste, you may add frozen raspberries or strawberries. This was enough for two or three children a day, but an adult could drink that much without hesitation.

Adults should drink:
Beet juice—3 parts
Carrot juice—2 parts
Celery root juice—12 part

If celery root juice cannot be obtained, the first 2 juices alone are very, very helpful. 5 ounces 2x daily.

The following herb tea will help to open the Portal Veins.

Mellilot
Calendula
St. John's Wort
Equal parts.

Leukemia is a serious disease, but there is *NO* fungus involvement.

Prof. Brauchle never lost a single case of a leukemia stricken child. Couldn't we try also? It takes only days to help.

How To Set the Tailbone

1

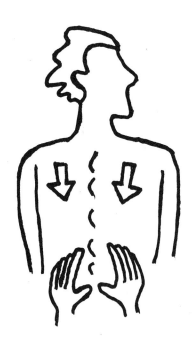

2

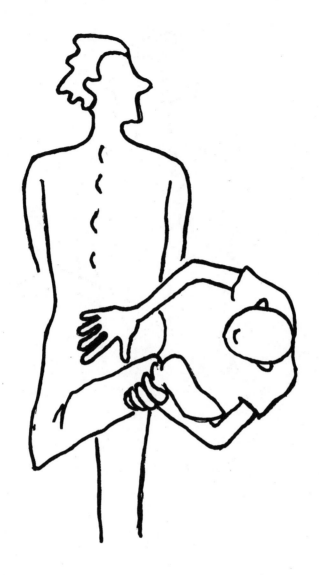

3

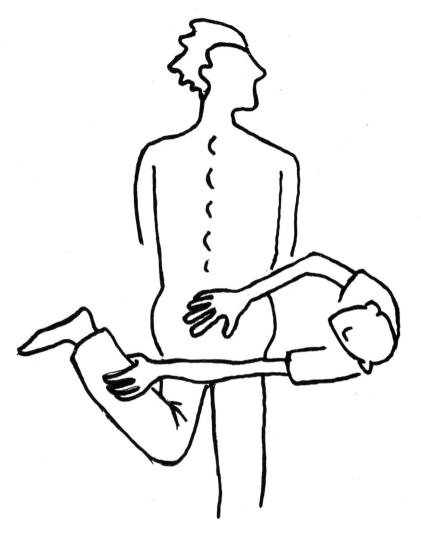

4

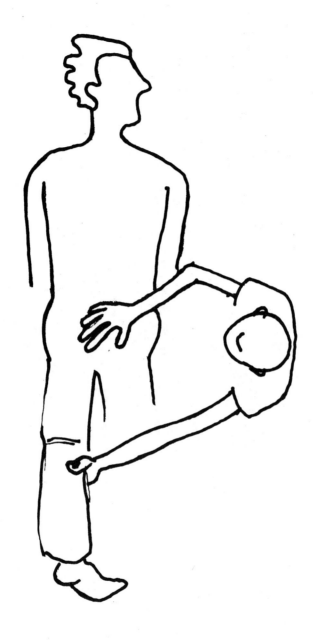

5

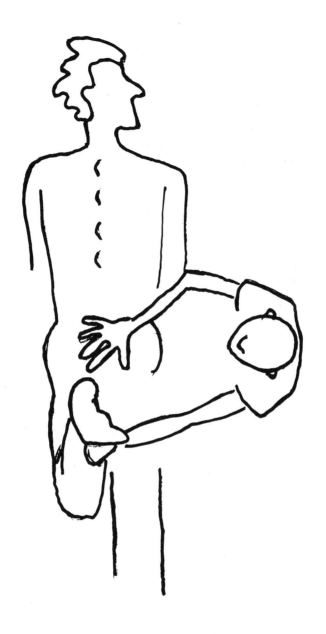

6

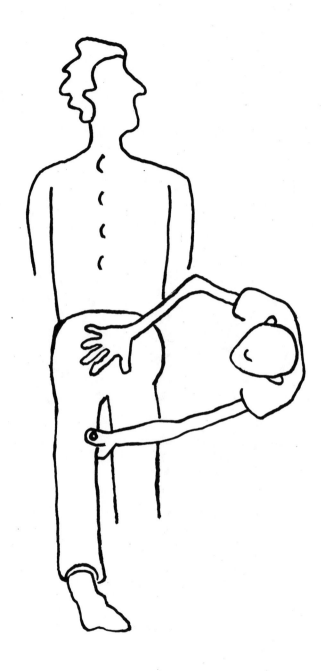

THE SPIRITUAL FACTOR IN THE
MANAGEMENT OF CANCER

This book would not be complete without the following chapter, the spiritual part in the management of cancer.

Cancer stricken people go through the following emotional upheavals:

disbelief
anger
despair
giving up

When you are diagnosed as having cancer, you will have a great disbelief.

"I have no pain."
"I am a little more tired."
"I am overworked."
"But I do not have cancer."

Always seek a second opinion. Suppress your thoughts and feelings of doom by saying to yourself, "All things are possible to him that believeth." (Mark 9:23).

After the verdict of the second physician, I suggest that you change your diet as outlined and also straighten out your thinking. From a possessive thinking switch over to a freedom of unpossessiveness.

You do not possess your children. They are God's children and you are allowed to help them and feed them for awhile but they are God's creation. So is your husband. The is an abundance of God's love and God's work. So are you, a joy to God. John 20:27 says, "Be not faithful but believing." Say constantly, "Yes Lord, I believe in the first stage of the discovery of cancer." Say these words constantly. As you believe in something, you also do something about it. And the change has to come in the wholeness of your being and the wholeness of your action.

When you arrive at the second stage, the stage of Anger, you will ask, Why Me? Why not my enemy. I have so much to do. Why has God given me this cross to bear. I honestly say good for you! Be angry, be mad, stamp your foot on the floor, kick your pillow, yell, run. Take the professional widespread concept, "you have cancer, you have to die," and rip it apart. Get ready to fight and fight well. Use the healthy power of your will! Will is an energy. Willpower is located in your forehead and next to it is the power of understanding. If you use willpower, you might come upon trouble; but with willpower comes understanding. The power of understanding goes into the depth of your being. Understanding goes to the intuitive power, which is God-centered. Will power and the power of understanding is expressed in the words, "not mine but Thy will be done." This is not a negative statement. Thy will O Lord is health, well-being, and happy accomplishments, so I will understand this and get well quickly to do His will on earth.

The third stage of your way downhill is despair. When you are in despair, your muscles contract and circulation is cut off. You start having pain. You think that this is the end of your life. Relax, relax. Ask for the power of strength and ask for the Divine Order of Christ. Your power of order is at your solar plexus. This solar plexus also is the vessel, The Golden Grail, through which new ideas, new inventions, new strength is arising. When this vessel is full of old junk, such as resentment, unforgiveness, disharmony, and negative emotions, the power of order cannot manifest. Clean out that stuff and start anew. As soon as you have cleared this vessel, Hope will enter. Where there is hope, life will enter. Where there is life, God holds your precious life in his hands and will give you strength, endurance, and love.

The last of the four stages is that one in which cancer patients will "give in." They sit there and wait for the hour to part from us. Oh dear beloved brother, dearest sister, only God knows the hour. We had a physician in class. He said, "I have seen miracles. I thought 'this breath is the last breath my fellowman is taking,' but it was not the last, but the first of a long life to come. Never give up."

My book "The Seven Spiritual Causes of Ill Health" will help you tremendously. On request, The Chapel of Miracles will send you healing prayers. Send handwriting and full name to:

Chapel of Miracles
7075 Valmont Road
Boulder, Colorado 80301

Pearls from the Bible for Healing

PSALM 3:1–9
> For with Thee is the fountain of life, in Thy light shall we see light.

PSALM 3
> But thou, O Lord, art a Shield for me; my glory, and the lifter up of my head.
> I cried unto the Lord with my voice, and He heard me—out of His Holy Hill Selah, Selah, Selah.

PROVERBS 17:22
> And ye shall serve the Lord Your God, and He shall bless thy bread and thy water. And He will take sickness away from the midst of thee.

ISAIAH 38–21
> For Isaiah had said
> Let me take a lump of figs and lay it for a plaster on the boil and he shall recover.

PROVERBS 24:13
> My son eat thou the honey because it is good, and the honeycomb which is sweet to thy taste.

When bleeding is present, read:

EZEKIEL 16–6, three times. The bleeding will stop.

> Three times in a row, three times a day, say:
> By his stripes, thou shall be healed.

You will be amazed what a relief this is to you when you have pain.